BLOOD SUGAR SOLUTION

FOR BEGINNERS

Empower Your Health: The Blood Sugar Diet for Lasting Change

Lori J. Carter

TABLE OF CONTENTS

INTRODUCTION

Welcome to the world of blood sugar management. In these pages, you'll discover a practical approach to improving your health and well-being through simple dietary changes and lifestyle adjustments. But before we delve into the details of the blood sugar diet solution, let me share with you a personal story that ignited my journey into this transformative path.

It was a regular visit to the doctor's office when I received news that would change my life forever. The blood test results revealed that my blood sugar levels were higher than they should be. It was a wake-up call, a stark reminder of the importance of taking charge of my health. Fear and uncertainty gripped me as I grappled with the implications of this diagnosis. But amidst the uncertainty, there was a glimmer of hope - the opportunity to make positive changes and reclaim control over my health.

Driven by a desire to regain vitality and vitality, I embarked on a journey to understand the intricacies of blood sugar management. I devoured every piece of information, from scientific studies to personal anecdotes, seeking clarity and guidance. Along the way, I experimented with various dietary approaches and lifestyle modifications, learning firsthand the profound impact they could have on blood sugar levels and overall well-being.

Through trial and error, I uncovered the principles of the blood sugar diet solution - a simple yet powerful framework for achieving optimal health and vitality. It's not about deprivation or strict rules but rather about making informed choices that nourish the body and support stable blood sugar levels. And now, I'm excited to share these insights with you, so you too can experience the transformative power of the blood sugar diet solution.

But this book is more than just a collection of information; it's a call to action. It's an invitation to take control of your health and embark on a journey of self-discovery and empowerment. So I urge you to dive into these pages with an open mind and a willingness to embrace change. Let's embark on this journey together, step by step, as we uncover the wonders of the blood sugar diet solution and unlock the door to a healthier, happier life.

Are you prepared to move forward in the direction of a more promising future? Let's embark on this journey together and discover the transformative power of the blood sugar diet solution. Your health and vitality await.

CHAPTER 1:

UNDERSTANDING BLOOD SUGAR

In the intricate symphony of human biology, blood sugar serves as a crucial note, harmonizing the energy flow essential for our body's function. Yet, what exactly is blood sugar, and why does it hold such paramount importance in our daily lives? Join me as we embark on a journey to demystify blood sugar, unraveling its essence, function, and profound implications for our health and well-being.

Understanding Blood Sugar: The Basics

At its essence, blood sugar, scientifically known as glucose, is a simple sugar molecule that courses through our bloodstream, akin to the lifeblood that sustains our bodily functions. It serves as the primary source of energy for our cells, fueling every aspect of our existence, from basic metabolic processes to the most intricate cognitive tasks.

My Personal Journey with Blood Sugar

Reflecting on my own journey, there was a pivotal moment that illuminated the significance of blood sugar in my life. During a routine health check, my physician delivered a sobering revelation: my blood sugar levels were higher than optimal, signaling a potential imbalance that warranted attention. This revelation sparked a profound curiosity within me, igniting a quest to comprehend the intricacies of blood sugar and its profound impact on our health.

The Digestive Symphony

The journey of blood sugar commences with the consumption of carbohydrates, which serve as its primary source. Carbohydrates, prevalent in a myriad of foods such as grains, fruits, and vegetables, undergo digestion in our gastrointestinal tract, where they are broken down into simpler sugars, including glucose. Once liberated, glucose traverses the intestinal wall and enters our bloodstream, where it becomes readily available to nourish our cells.

The Role of Insulin: A Gatekeeper of Energy

Yet, glucose's journey to cellular sustenance is not a solitary endeavor; it relies upon the assistance of a vital hormone known as insulin. Produced by the pancreas, insulin serves as the gatekeeper of energy, facilitating the entry of glucose into our cells. Through a finely orchestrated dance, insulin binds to receptors on cell membranes, initiating a cascade of events that culminate in the uptake of glucose—a process essential for cellular vitality and function.

Balancing Act: Maintaining Glucose Homeostasis

Maintaining optimal blood sugar levels is paramount for our health, as deviations from the norm can yield profound consequences. When blood sugar levels soar beyond the body's threshold, a state known as hyperglycemia ensues, characterized by symptoms such as increased thirst, frequent urination, fatigue, and blurred vision. Conversely, plunging blood sugar levels, or hypoglycemia, can induce symptoms ranging from shakiness and confusion to seizures and loss of consciousness.

Navigating the Ebb and Flow

Our blood sugar levels undergo a perpetual ebb and flow, modulated by an array of factors including dietary intake, physical activity, stress, and hormonal fluctuations. While these fluctuations are a natural facet of human physiology, for some individuals—particularly those grappling with conditions such as diabetes—maintaining stable blood sugar levels may necessitate vigilant monitoring and management.

The Significance of Awareness

Awareness serves as a cornerstone in the quest for blood sugar equilibrium. By understanding the nuances of blood sugar regulation and its profound implications for our health, we empower ourselves to make informed choices that nurture our well-being. Whether through mindful dietary selections, regular physical activity, stress management techniques, or vigilant monitoring of blood sugar levels, each action plays a pivotal role in safeguarding our metabolic harmony.

In essence, blood sugar stands as an indispensable component of our physiological tapestry, intricately woven into the fabric of our existence. Through a deeper comprehension of its essence and function, we unlock the keys to optimal health and vitality, traversing a path illuminated by knowledge, awareness, and proactive engagement. As we continue our exploration into the realm of blood sugar, let us embark upon this odyssey with curiosity, reverence, and a steadfast commitment to holistic well-being.

How the Body Regulates Blood Sugar Levels

In the intricate dance of human physiology, maintaining optimal blood sugar levels is akin to orchestrating a finely tuned symphony. It requires a delicate balance of hormones, enzymes, and cellular processes working in harmony to ensure that our body has a steady supply of energy while avoiding the perils of excessive or deficient blood sugar levels. Join me as we delve into the fascinating mechanisms through which the body regulates blood sugar levels, exploring its intricacies and implications for our health and well-being.

Understanding Blood Sugar Regulation: An Overview

Before we delve into the intricate mechanisms of blood sugar regulation, let's take a moment to grasp the overarching principles governing this process. Blood sugar regulation is a dynamic and tightly controlled process that involves multiple organs, hormones, and cellular signaling pathways. Its primary goal is to maintain blood sugar levels within a narrow range, ensuring an adequate supply of energy to meet the body's demands while avoiding the detrimental effects of either hypoglycemia, which is low blood sugar, or hyperglycemia, which is elevated blood sugar.

My Personal Journey with Blood Sugar Regulation

Reflecting on my own journey, I recall the profound impact that fluctuations in blood sugar levels had on my health and well-being. From the highs of hyperglycemia-induced fatigue and thirst to the lows of hypoglycemic episodes characterized by dizziness and confusion, I experienced firsthand the importance of maintaining stable blood sugar levels. It was this personal journey that fueled my curiosity and drove me to explore the intricate mechanisms through which the body regulates blood sugar.

The Role of Hormones: Insulin and Glucagon

At the heart of blood sugar regulation lie two pivotal hormones: insulin and glucagon. Produced by the pancreas—a gland located behind the stomach—these hormones work in tandem to maintain blood sugar homeostasis.

1. Insulin: The Gatekeeper of Glucose

Insulin facilitates the entry of glucose into cells, which is a key mechanism by which blood sugar levels are reduced. When blood sugar levels rise—such as after a meal rich in carbohydrates—specialized cells in the pancreas called beta cells release insulin into the bloodstream. Insulin then binds to receptors on the surface of target cells, signaling them to take up glucose from the bloodstream and convert it into energy or store it for future use. This process helps reduce blood sugar levels, ensuring that excess glucose is efficiently utilized by the body.

2. Glucagon: Mobilizing Stored Energy

In contrast to insulin, glucagon acts to raise blood sugar levels when they fall too low. Produced by alpha cells in the pancreas, glucagon stimulates the breakdown of glycogen—a stored form of glucose found in the liver and muscles—into glucose, which is released into the bloodstream. This process, known as glycogenolysis, helps replenish blood sugar levels during periods of fasting or increased energy demand, ensuring a steady supply of glucose to fuel the body's needs.

The Liver: A Key Player in Blood Sugar Regulation

The liver plays a pivotal role in blood sugar regulation, serving as a storage site for glycogen and a primary source of glucose production. In response to hormonal signals such as insulin and glucagon, the liver adjusts its glucose output to maintain blood sugar levels within a narrow range.

Muscle and Fat Cells: Sites of Glucose Utilization and Storage

Muscle and fat cells also contribute to blood sugar regulation by absorbing glucose from the bloodstream in response to insulin. Once inside these cells, glucose can be used for energy production or stored as glycogen (in muscle cells) or triglycerides (in fat cells) for later use.

The Role of the Brain: A Glucose-Dependent Organ

The brain, despite comprising only about 2% of our body weight, is highly dependent on glucose as its primary source of energy. Maintaining stable blood sugar levels is essential for ensuring an adequate supply of glucose to the brain, as fluctuations can impair cognitive function and lead to symptoms such as confusion, dizziness, and fainting.

Stress Hormones: A Double-Edged Sword

In times of stress or perceived danger, the body releases stress hormones such as cortisol and adrenaline, which can temporarily raise blood sugar levels. While this response is essential for mobilizing energy to cope with stressful situations, chronic stress or prolonged elevation of stress hormones can disrupt blood sugar regulation and contribute to insulin resistance and metabolic dysfunction.

The Role of Exercise: Enhancing Insulin Sensitivity

Regular physical activity plays a crucial role in blood sugar regulation by improving insulin sensitivity and enhancing glucose uptake by muscles. Exercise helps lower blood sugar levels by increasing the efficiency of insulin action, making it easier for cells to absorb glucose from the bloodstream and utilize it for energy production.

Dietary Factors: Balancing Carbohydrates and Fiber

Dietary choices also play a significant role in blood sugar regulation. Consuming a balanced diet rich in complex carbohydrates, fiber, and protein can help stabilize blood sugar levels by promoting slow and steady glucose absorption. In contrast, excessive consumption of refined carbohydrates and sugary foods can lead to rapid spikes in blood sugar levels, followed by crashes that may contribute to insulin resistance and metabolic dysfunction.

Types of Carbohydrates and Their Effect on Blood Sugar

In the realm of nutrition, carbohydrates reign supreme as the primary source of energy for our bodies. From the humble potato to the indulgent slice of cake, carbohydrates come in a myriad of forms, each with its unique impact on blood sugar levels. Join me as we explore the diverse landscape of carbohydrates, unraveling their nuances and understanding how they influence our blood sugar.

Understanding Carbohydrates: The Basics

Before delving into the intricacies of different carbohydrate types, let's establish a foundational understanding of what carbohydrates are. Carbohydrates are macronutrients found in a variety of foods, including grains, fruits, vegetables, legumes, and dairy products. They consist of carbon, hydrogen, and oxygen atoms arranged in various structures, from simple sugars to complex starches and fibers.

My Personal Journey with Carbohydrates

Reflecting on my own dietary journey, I recall the profound impact that different types of carbohydrates had on my blood sugar levels and overall well-being. From the rapid spike in energy followed by a crash induced by sugary snacks to the sustained energy and satiety provided by fiber-rich whole grains and vegetables, my experiences underscored the importance of choosing carbohydrates wisely.

Simple Carbohydrates: The Quick Energy Fix

One or two sugar molecules make up simple carbohydrates, also referred to as sugars, which are swiftly absorbed and processed into the bloodstream, causing sharp rises in blood sugar levels. Common sources of simple carbohydrates include table sugar, honey, syrups, fruit juices, and refined grains like white bread and pasta.

Effect on Blood Sugar: The Sugar Rollercoaster

Consuming foods high in simple carbohydrates can lead to a rapid increase in blood sugar levels, followed by a subsequent crash as insulin levels rise to shuttle glucose into cells. This rollercoaster effect can leave you feeling lethargic, hungry, and irritable, prompting further cravings for sugary snacks and perpetuating the cycle of blood sugar fluctuations.

Complex Carbohydrates: The Sustained Energy Source

In contrast to simple carbohydrates, complex carbohydrates consist of long chains of sugar molecules and take longer to digest and absorb, resulting in a slower and more sustained release of glucose into the bloodstream. Common sources of complex carbohydrates include whole grains, legumes, vegetables, and fruits.

Effect on Blood Sugar: The Steady Stream

Consuming foods rich in complex carbohydrates can help stabilize blood sugar levels by providing a steady stream of glucose to fuel your body's energy needs. Unlike simple carbohydrates, which cause rapid spikes and crashes in blood sugar, complex carbohydrates promote sustained energy and satiety, helping you feel fuller for longer and reducing cravings for sugary snacks.

Fiber: The Unsung Hero of Carbohydrates

Fiber, a type of complex carbohydrate found in plant foods, plays a crucial role in blood sugar regulation and overall health. Unlike other carbohydrates, fiber is not digested or absorbed by the body but instead passes through the digestive tract relatively intact, adding bulk to stools and promoting regularity.

Effect on Blood Sugar: The Blood Sugar Buffer

Fiber acts as a natural blood sugar buffer, slowing the absorption of glucose and preventing rapid spikes in blood sugar levels. Foods high in fiber, such as whole grains, fruits, vegetables, legumes, and nuts, can help improve insulin sensitivity, reduce the risk of type 2 diabetes, and promote weight management.

Glycemic Index: The Measure of Carbohydrate Impact

Foods containing carbohydrates are ranked on a scale called the glycemic index (GI) according to how they affect blood sugar levels. Foods with a high GI are rapidly digested and absorbed, causing rapid spikes in blood sugar, whole foods with a low GI are digested and absorbed more slowly, leading to a slow rise in blood glucose levels.

Effect on Blood Sugar: Making Informed Choices

By choosing carbohydrates with a low or moderate GI, such as whole grains, legumes, fruits, and vegetables, you can help stabilize blood sugar levels, improve insulin sensitivity, and reduce the risk of long-term conditions such heart disease and type 2 diabetes. Additionally, pairing carbohydrates with protein, healthy fats, and fiber-rich foods can further mitigate their impact on blood sugar levels.

In conclusion, understanding the different types of carbohydrates and their effect on blood sugar is essential for making informed dietary choices and promoting overall health and well-being. By opting for complex carbohydrates rich in fiber and nutrients and minimizing consumption of simple carbohydrates, you can support stable blood sugar levels, sustained energy, and long-term vitality. So, let's embark on a journey of carbohydrate exploration, embracing the diversity of flavors and textures that nature has to offer while nourishing our bodies and nurturing our health.

Glycemic Index and Glycemic Load Explained

Understanding how different foods affect our blood sugar levels is crucial for maintaining overall health and well-being. Two key concepts that play a significant role in this understanding are the glycemic index (GI) and glycemic load (GL). In this section, we will explore these concepts in detail, drawing from both scientific knowledge and personal experiences to provide clarity on how they impact our dietary choices and health outcomes.

Understanding Glycemic Index (GI): A Measure of Blood Sugar Response

Foods containing carbohydrates are ranked on the glycemic index according to how quickly their blood sugar levels rise after ingestion. Foods with a high GI cause a rapid spike in blood sugar, while those with a low GI lead to a slower, more gradual increase. The GI scale ranges from 0 to 100, with pure glucose having a GI of 100.

Personal Experience with Glycemic Index

Reflecting on my own journey, I vividly recall the impact that understanding GI had on my dietary choices and overall well-being. I noticed that when I consumed foods with a high GI, such as sugary snacks or refined carbohydrates, I experienced a quick surge in energy followed by a crash. This rollercoaster effect left me feeling tired and irritable, prompting me to seek out alternatives that would provide more stable energy levels throughout the day.

How Glycemic Index is Determined

The GI of a food is determined by feeding a group of people a portion of the food containing a standardized amount of carbohydrate and then measuring their blood sugar response over the next few hours. The area under the curve of the blood sugar response is compared to that of pure glucose, and the resulting value is expressed as a percentage of glucose's effect.

Examples of Foods with Different Glycemic Index Values

1. Low GI foods: Legumes, non-starchy vegetables, whole grains, nuts, and seeds.

2. Medium GI foods: Oatmeal, brown rice, whole wheat bread, sweet potatoes.

3. High GI foods: White bread, white rice, sugary cereals, baked goods, sugary beverages.

Understanding Glycemic Load (GL): Accounting for Portion Size

While the glycemic index provides valuable information about how individual foods affect blood sugar levels, it does not consider the quantity of carbohydrates consumed. This is where the concept of glycemic load comes into play. Glycemic load takes into account both the quality and quantity of carbohydrates in a serving of food, providing a more accurate measure of its impact on blood sugar levels.

Personal Insights into Glycemic Load

In my own experience, I found that considering both GI and portion size was essential for managing blood sugar levels effectively. By choosing foods with a lower glycemic load and moderating portion sizes, I was able to achieve more stable energy levels and reduce cravings for sugary snacks.

How to Calculate Glycemic Load

Glycemic load is calculated by multiplying the glycemic index of a food by the amount of carbohydrate it contains per serving and dividing by 100. This calculation provides a numerical value that indicates the overall impact of a food on blood sugar levels.

Incorporating Glycemic Index and Glycemic Load into Everyday Life

Incorporating GI and GL into your daily diet can be straightforward and practical. Here are some tips to help you make informed choices:

1. Choose whole, unprocessed foods: Whole grains, fruits, vegetables, legumes, nuts, and seeds tend to have lower GI and GL values compared to processed foods.

2. Opt for smaller portion sizes: Even low GI foods can contribute to blood sugar spikes if consumed in large quantities, so be mindful of portion sizes.

3. Balance your meals: Pair high GI foods with protein, healthy fats, and fiber-rich foods to slow down the absorption of carbohydrates and stabilize blood sugar levels.

In summary, understanding the glycemic index and glycemic load of foods can empower you to make informed dietary choices that promote stable blood sugar levels and overall health. By choosing foods with a lower GI and GL and considering portion sizes, you can optimize your energy levels, reduce cravings, and support long-term well-being. So, let's continue to explore the fascinating world of nutrition, armed with knowledge and a commitment to nurturing our bodies from the inside out.

CHAPTER 2:

THE BLOOD SUGAR DIET PLAN

Embarking on a journey toward better health often involves understanding the principles that govern our dietary choices. In the realm of blood sugar management, adopting a strategic approach can yield profound benefits for overall well-being. Join me as we explore the fundamental principles of the Blood Sugar Diet, drawing from both scientific knowledge and personal experience to illuminate the path toward optimal health.

Understanding the Blood Sugar Diet: A Holistic Approach

The Blood Sugar Diet is more than just a dietary regimen; it's a comprehensive lifestyle approach aimed at stabilizing blood sugar levels, promoting weight loss, and enhancing overall health. At its core, this approach emphasizes mindful eating, balanced nutrition, regular physical activity, and stress management—all essential components for achieving metabolic harmony and vitality.

My Personal Experience with the Blood Sugar Diet

Reflecting on my own journey, I recall the transformative impact that embracing the principles of the Blood Sugar Diet had on my health and well-being. By adopting a mindful approach to eating, prioritizing nutrient-dense foods, and incorporating regular exercise into my routine, I experienced significant improvements in my energy levels, mood, and overall vitality. This personal journey fueled my passion for sharing the principles of the Blood Sugar Diet with others, inspiring them to embark on their own paths toward better health.

Principle 1: Embrace Whole, Nutrient-Dense Foods

At the heart of the Blood Sugar Diet lies a focus on whole, nutrient-dense foods that nourish the body and support optimal health. These foods include fresh fruits and vegetables, whole grains, lean proteins, healthy fats, and legumes—each brimming with essential vitamins, minerals, antioxidants, and fiber. By prioritizing these nutrient-rich choices, we provide our bodies with the building blocks they need to thrive while minimizing the intake of processed and refined foods that can disrupt blood sugar balance.

Principle 2: Balance Macronutrients for Sustained Energy

Achieving a balanced intake of macronutrients—carbohydrates, proteins, and fats—is key to supporting stable blood sugar levels and sustained energy throughout the day. While carbohydrates serve as the body's primary source of energy, pairing them with protein, healthy fats, and fiber-rich foods can help slow down their absorption, preventing rapid spikes and crashes in blood sugar. This balanced approach promotes satiety, reduces cravings, and supports overall metabolic health.

Principle 3: Monitor Portion Sizes and Timing

Portion control and meal timing play crucial roles in blood sugar management and weight regulation. By being mindful of portion sizes and spacing meals evenly throughout the day, we can prevent excessive caloric intake and minimize fluctuations in blood sugar levels. Additionally, incorporating smaller, more frequent meals and snacks can help maintain energy levels and prevent overeating, supporting a steady supply of nutrients to fuel our activities.

Principle 4: Choose Low-Glycemic Foods

Adopting a diet rich in low-glycemic foods—those that have minimal impact on blood sugar levels—can further support blood sugar balance and metabolic health. These foods include non-starchy vegetables, legumes, whole grains, nuts, seeds, and some fruits, which are digested and absorbed slowly, leading to a gradual rise in blood sugar. By incorporating these nutrient-dense choices into our meals and snacks, we can promote satiety, enhance insulin sensitivity, and reduce the risk of chronic diseases.

Principle 5: Prioritize Hydration and Mindful Eating

Hydration and mindful eating are integral components of the Blood Sugar Diet, supporting digestion, satiety, and overall well-being. Drinking an adequate amount of water throughout the day helps maintain proper hydration levels, supports metabolic function, and may help curb cravings for sugary beverages. Additionally, practicing mindful eating—such as savoring each bite, paying attention to hunger and fullness cues, and avoiding distractions—can promote a deeper connection with food and foster healthier eating habits.

Principle 6: Incorporate Regular Physical Activity

Physical activity is a cornerstone of the Blood Sugar Diet, promoting cardiovascular health, weight management, and insulin sensitivity. Engaging in regular exercise—whether it's brisk walking, cycling, strength training, or yoga—helps lower blood sugar levels, improve glucose utilization, and enhance overall fitness. Aim for at least 150 minutes of moderate-intensity exercise per week, along with strength training exercises two or more days per week, to reap the full benefits of physical activity.

Principle 7: Practice Stress Management and Self-Care

Stress management and self-care are essential components of the Blood Sugar Diet, as chronic stress can disrupt blood sugar balance and contribute to weight gain and metabolic dysfunction. Incorporating relaxation techniques such as deep breathing, meditation, yoga, and mindfulness can help reduce stress levels, improve mood, and support overall well-being. Additionally, prioritizing adequate sleep, nurturing social connections, and engaging in activities that bring joy and fulfillment can further promote resilience and vitality.

Incorporating the Principles into Daily Life

Incorporating the principles of the Blood Sugar Diet into daily life can be simple and practical with a few key strategies:

1. Plan and prepare meals ahead of time to ensure access to nutrient-dense options.

2. Keep healthy snacks on hand to prevent impulsive choices when hunger strikes.

3. Experiment with new recipes and flavor combinations to keep meals exciting and satisfying.

4. Stay active throughout the day by incorporating movement into daily routines, such as taking the stairs or going for a walk during breaks.

5. Prioritize self-care activities that nourish the mind, body, and spirit, such as spending time in nature, practicing gratitude, and cultivating meaningful relationships.

In conclusion, the principles of the Blood Sugar Diet offer a roadmap to optimal health and vitality, emphasizing whole, nutrient-dense foods, balanced nutrition, regular physical activity, and stress management. By embracing these principles and making mindful choices in our daily lives, we can support stable blood sugar levels, promote weight loss, and enhance overall well-being. So, let's embark on this journey together, armed with knowledge, inspiration, and a commitment to nurturing our bodies and minds from the inside out.

Creating Your Blood Sugar Diet Meal Plan

Embarking on the journey of the Blood Sugar Diet requires a strategic approach to meal planning. Crafting a personalized meal plan that aligns with the principles of balanced nutrition, mindful eating, and blood sugar management is essential for achieving optimal health and well-being. In this chapter, we will delve into the process of creating your Blood Sugar Diet meal plan, drawing insights from both scientific knowledge and personal experiences to guide you on your path to success.

Understanding the Importance of Meal Planning

Meal planning is a cornerstone of the Blood Sugar Diet, providing structure and organization to your dietary habits. By planning your meals ahead of time, you can ensure access to nutritious options, prevent impulsive choices, and support blood sugar balance throughout the day. Additionally, meal planning can save time and money, reduce food waste, and alleviate the stress of deciding what to eat on a daily basis.

My Personal Experience with Meal Planning

Reflecting on my own journey, I recognize the transformative impact that meal planning had on my ability to adhere to the Blood Sugar Diet and achieve my health goals. By taking the time to plan and prepare my meals in advance, I found that I was better equipped to make mindful choices, resist temptation, and maintain consistency in my dietary habits. This personalized approach allowed me to align my meals with the principles of the Blood Sugar Diet while catering to my individual tastes and preferences.

Steps to Creating Your Blood Sugar Diet Meal Plan

1. Set Clear Goals: Before creating your meal plan, take some time to define your health and wellness goals. Whether you're aiming to stabilize blood sugar levels, lose weight, or improve overall vitality, clarifying your objectives will help inform your meal planning process.

2. Assess Your Nutritional Needs: Consider factors such as age, gender, activity level, and any specific dietary requirements or restrictions when determining your nutritional needs. Aim to include a balance of macronutrients—carbohydrates, proteins, and fats—in each meal to support stable blood sugar levels and sustained energy throughout the day.

3. Choose Nutrient-Dense Foods: Base your meal plan around whole, nutrient-dense foods that provide essential vitamins, minerals, antioxidants, and fiber. Incorporate a variety of fruits, vegetables,

whole grains, lean proteins, healthy fats, and legumes to ensure a well-rounded and nourishing diet.

4. Balance Your Macronutrients: Aim to include a source of protein, healthy fat, and fiber-rich carbohydrates in each meal to promote satiety, stabilize blood sugar levels, and support overall metabolic health. Experiment with different combinations and portion sizes to find what works best for you.

5. Consider Glycemic Index and Glycemic Load: When selecting carbohydrates for your meal plan, prioritize low-glycemic options that have minimal impact on blood sugar levels. Incorporating foods with a lower glycemic index and glycemic load, such as non-starchy vegetables, whole grains, and legumes, can help support blood sugar balance and reduce the risk of insulin resistance.

6. Plan Ahead and Prep: Take time each week to plan your meals, create a shopping list, and prep ingredients in advance. Batch cooking and meal prepping can streamline the process and make it easier to stick to your meal plan, especially during busy weekdays.

7. Stay Flexible and Adapt: While having a meal plan in place is beneficial, it's important to remain flexible and adaptable to changes in schedule,

preferences, and circumstances. Don't be afraid to modify your meal plan as needed and experiment with new recipes and ingredients to keep things interesting and enjoyable.

Sample Blood Sugar Diet Meal Plan

To help you get started, here's a sample Blood Sugar Diet meal plan for a day:

Breakfast:

1. Feta and spinach omelet served with whole grain bread.

2. Green tea or black coffee

Mid-Morning Snack:

Greek yogurt with sliced strawberries and almonds.

Lunch:

1. Grilled salmon salad with mixed greens, cherry tomatoes, cucumbers, and avocado.

2. Balsamic vinaigrette dressing.

Afternoon Snack:

Carrot sticks with hummus.

Dinner:

1. Quinoa and vegetable stir-fry with tofu or chicken.

2. Steamed broccoli on the side.

3. Herbal tea or infused water for hydration.

Evening Snack (Optional):

Apple slices with almond butter.

In summary, creating your Blood Sugar Diet meal plan is a personalized and empowering process that involves setting clear goals, assessing your nutritional needs, and making mindful choices about the foods you consume. By prioritizing whole, nutrient-dense foods, balancing macronutrients, and incorporating low-glycemic options, you can support stable blood sugar levels, promote weight loss, and enhance overall vitality. So, take the time to plan and prepare your meals with intention, and let your meal plan serve as a guide on your journey to optimal health and well-being.

Sample Meal Plans and Recipes

Crafting a Blood Sugar Diet meal plan is a foundational step towards achieving optimal health and well-being. By incorporating nutrient-dense foods, balancing macronutrients, and prioritizing low-glycemic options, you can support stable blood sugar levels and promote overall vitality. In this chapter, we will explore sample meal plans and recipes to inspire you on your journey to better health, drawing insights from both scientific knowledge and personal experiences to guide you towards delicious and nourishing meals.

Introduction to Meal Planning

Meal planning is a proactive approach to healthy eating that involves thoughtful consideration of the foods you consume throughout the day. By taking the time to plan your meals in advance, you can ensure access to nutritious options, prevent impulsive choices, and support blood sugar balance. Whether you're aiming to stabilize blood sugar levels, lose weight, or improve overall well-being, meal planning can serve as a valuable tool in achieving your health goals.

My Personal Experience with Meal Planning

Reflecting on my own journey, I recognize the transformative impact that meal planning had on my ability to adhere to the Blood Sugar Diet and achieve my health goals. By incorporating nutrient-dense foods, balancing macronutrients, and prioritizing low-glycemic options, I was able to support stable blood sugar levels and promote overall vitality. This personalized approach allowed me to align my meals with the principles of the Blood Sugar Diet while catering to my individual tastes and preferences.

Sample Meal Plan 1: Balanced Breakfast

Breakfast:

Spinach and Mushroom Frittata

Ingredients:

1. 4 eggs

2. 1 cup spinach, chopped

3. 1/2 cup mushrooms, sliced

4. 1/4 cup onion, diced

5. 1/4 cup feta cheese, crumbled

6. Salt and pepper to taste

Instructions:

1. Preheat the oven to 375°F (190°C).

2. In a bowl, whisk together eggs, spinach, mushrooms, onion, and feta cheese. Season with salt and pepper.

3. Pour the mixture into a greased oven-safe skillet and bake for 15-20 minutes until the eggs are set and the top is golden brown.

4. Slice into wedges and serve hot.

Mid-Morning Snack:

Greek Yogurt Parfait

Ingredients:

1. 1/2 cup Greek yogurt

2. 1/4 cup mixed berries (strawberries, blueberries, raspberries)

3. 1 tablespoon almonds, chopped

4. 1 teaspoon honey (optional)

Sample Meal Plan 2: Wholesome Lunch

Lunch:

Quinoa Salad with Chickpeas and Avocado

Ingredients:

1. 1 cup cooked quinoa

2. 1/2 cup chickpeas, drained and rinsed

3. 1/2 avocado, diced

4. 1/4 cup cherry tomatoes, halved

5. 1/4 cup cucumber, diced

6. 2 tablespoons fresh parsley, chopped

7. 1 tablespoon olive oil

8. 1 tablespoon lemon juice

9. Salt and pepper to taste

Instructions:

1. In a large bowl, combine cooked quinoa, chickpeas, avocado, cherry tomatoes, cucumber, and parsley.

2. Drizzle with olive oil and lemon juice. To taste, add salt and pepper for seasoning.

3. Gently toss to mix, then serve cold or at room temperature.

Afternoon Snack:

Carrot Sticks with Hummus

Ingredients:

1. 2 medium carrots, cut into sticks

2. 1/4 cup hummus

Sample Meal Plan 3: Nutrient-Rich Dinner

Dinner:

Grilled Salmon with Asparagus and Quinoa

Ingredients:

1. 2 salmon filets

2. 1 bunch asparagus, trimmed

3. 1 cup cooked quinoa

4. 1 tablespoon olive oil

5. 1 tablespoon lemon juice

6. Salt and pepper to taste

Instructions:

1. Preheat the grill to medium-high heat.

2. Salmon filets are seasoned with salt, pepper, lemon juice, and olive oil.

3. Place salmon filets and asparagus spears on the grill. Cook for 4-5 minutes per side until salmon is cooked through and asparagus is tender.

4. Serve grilled salmon and asparagus with cooked quinoa on the side.

Evening Snack:

Apple Slices with Almond Butter

Ingredients:

1. 1 medium apple, sliced

2. 2 tablespoons almond butter

In summary, crafting a Blood Sugar Diet meal plan involves thoughtful consideration of nutrient-dense foods, balanced macronutrients, and low-glycemic options to support stable blood sugar levels and overall well-being. By incorporating delicious and nourishing recipes like the ones provided above, you can create meals that not only taste great but also promote optimal health and vitality. So, take the time to plan your meals with intention, and let your meal plan serve as a guide on your journey to better health.

CHAPTER 3:

LIFESTYLE STRATEGIES FOR BLOOD SUGAR MANAGEMENT

You've unlocked the secrets of blood sugar balance, understanding the internal dance between food and your body. Now, it's time to translate that knowledge into action! This chapter equips you with powerful lifestyle strategies – your personal toolbox for maintaining healthy blood sugar levels. We'll delve into the magic of movement, explore the mindful plate, and discover how stress management becomes your secret weapon. Imagine a life fueled by steady energy, vibrant health, and a newfound confidence in your ability to manage your blood sugar. Let's embark on this empowering journey together!

Exercise Is Essential for Blood Sugar Management

Physical activity plays a crucial role in blood sugar control and overall health. Incorporating regular exercise into your routine can help regulate blood sugar levels, improve insulin sensitivity, and reduce the risk of developing type 2 diabetes. In this chapter, we will explore the importance of physical activity in blood sugar control, drawing from both scientific research and personal experiences to highlight its profound benefits and provide practical tips for incorporating exercise into your daily life.

Understanding the Link Between Physical Activity and Blood Sugar Control

Physical activity has a direct impact on blood sugar levels by increasing the uptake of glucose into cells, where it is used for energy production. During exercise, muscles become more sensitive to insulin, allowing them to take up glucose from the bloodstream more efficiently. This helps to lower blood sugar levels and reduce the risk of hyperglycemia, or high blood sugar.

My Personal Experience

Reflecting on my own journey, I've experienced firsthand the positive effects of regular physical activity on blood sugar control. By incorporating exercise into my daily routine, I've been able to maintain stable blood sugar levels, improve my overall health, and reduce my risk of developing diabetes. These personal experiences have reinforced the importance of physical activity in managing blood sugar and inspired me to share these insights with others.

Benefits of Physical Activity for Blood Sugar Control

1. Improves Insulin Sensitivity: Regular physical activity helps to improve insulin sensitivity, allowing cells to more effectively respond to insulin and uptake glucose from the bloodstream. Insulin resistance is a major contributing factor to the onset of type 2 diabetes, and this can help avoid it.

2. Lowers Blood Sugar Levels: Exercise promotes the utilization of glucose by muscles for energy production, leading to a decrease in blood sugar levels. This helps to prevent spikes in blood sugar and reduces the risk of complications associated with hyperglycemia.

3. Aids in Weight Management: Physical activity plays a crucial role in weight management by helping to burn calories and maintain a healthy body weight. Excess body weight is a risk factor for insulin resistance and type 2 diabetes, making regular exercise an important component of blood sugar control.

4. Reduces Cardiovascular Risk: Regular physical activity has cardiovascular benefits, including

lowering blood pressure, improving cholesterol levels, and reducing the risk of heart disease. People with diabetes are at higher risk of cardiovascular complications, making exercise an essential part of overall risk reduction.

5. Promotes Overall Health and Well-Being: In addition to its effects on blood sugar control, exercise has numerous benefits for overall health and well-being. It can improve mood, reduce stress, increase energy levels, and enhance quality of life.

Types of Physical Activity for Blood Sugar Control

1. Aerobic Exercise: Aerobic exercise, also known as cardio, involves activities that increase your heart rate and breathing, such as walking, jogging, cycling, swimming, and dancing. Try to get in at least 150 minutes a week, spread across multiple days, of moderate-intensity aerobic exercise.

2. Strength Training: Strength training, or resistance exercise, involves working your muscles against resistance to build strength and endurance. This can include activities such as weightlifting, bodyweight exercises, and resistance band workouts. Aim to

include strength training exercises two or more days per week, targeting all major muscle groups.

3. Flexibility and Balance Exercises: Flexibility and balance exercises help to improve range of motion, reduce the risk of injury, and enhance overall mobility. Examples include yoga, tai chi, and stretching exercises. Incorporate these activities into your routine to improve flexibility and balance.

Practical Tips for Incorporating Physical Activity into Your Routine

1. Start Slowly: If you've never worked out before or haven't been active in a while, begin with small steps and progressively increase the duration and intensity of your exercises. Listen to your body and choose activities that you enjoy and feel comfortable with.

2. Find Activities You Enjoy: Physical activity doesn't have to be boring or monotonous. Find activities that you enjoy and look forward to, whether it's dancing, hiking, playing sports, or taking group fitness classes. The more enjoyable and engaging the activity, the more likely you are to stick with it.

3. Make It a Habit: Schedule regular exercise sessions into your weekly routine, just like you would any other appointment or commitment. Consistency is key to reaping the benefits of physical activity for blood sugar control.

4. Stay Active Throughout the Day: Look for opportunities to incorporate physical activity into your daily life, such as taking the stairs instead of the elevator, walking or biking to work, or doing household chores and gardening. Every little bit of movement counts toward improving blood sugar control and overall health.

5. Set Realistic Goals: Set realistic and achievable goals for your physical activity routine, whether it's increasing the duration of your workouts, improving your strength and endurance, or participating in a specific event or challenge. Celebrate your progress along the way and adjust your goals as needed.

In conclusion, physical activity is a cornerstone of blood sugar control and overall health. By incorporating regular exercise into your routine, you can improve insulin sensitivity, lower blood sugar levels, manage your weight, reduce cardiovascular risk, and enhance your overall well-being. Whether it's aerobic exercise, strength training, flexibility and balance exercises, or simply staying active throughout the day, find activities that you enjoy and make them a way of life

Stress Management Techniques for Stable Blood Sugar

Managing stress is essential for maintaining stable blood sugar levels and overall well-being. Chronic stress can lead to fluctuations in blood sugar, insulin resistance, and increased risk of developing type 2 diabetes. In this chapter, we will explore various stress management techniques that can help you maintain stable blood sugar, drawing from both scientific research and personal experiences to provide practical insights and strategies.

Recognizing How Stress Affects Blood Sugar

Stress triggers the release of hormones such as cortisol and adrenaline, which can raise blood sugar levels by stimulating the liver to release glucose into the bloodstream. Additionally, stress can affect eating habits and lead to emotional eating or cravings for high-sugar, high-fat foods, further contributing to blood sugar fluctuations. Chronic stress can also impair insulin sensitivity, making it more challenging to regulate blood sugar levels over time.

My Personal Experience

Reflecting on my own journey, I've experienced firsthand the effects of stress on blood sugar control. During periods of heightened stress, I noticed fluctuations in my blood sugar levels and struggled to maintain stable glucose readings. However, by incorporating stress management techniques into my routine, I was able to mitigate these effects and better manage my blood sugar. These personal experiences have underscored the importance of stress management in maintaining overall health and well-being.

Stress Management Techniques

1. Deep Breathing Exercises: Deep breathing exercises can help activate the body's relaxation response, counteracting the effects of stress on blood sugar. Practice deep breathing by inhaling deeply through your nose, filling your lungs with air, and exhaling slowly through your mouth. Repeat this several times, paying attention to each breath and giving yourself permission to unwind.

2. Mindfulness Meditation: Focusing your attention on the current moment without passing judgment is the practice of mindfulness meditation. Regular practice of mindfulness meditation can help reduce

stress levels, improve emotional regulation, and enhance overall well-being. Locate a peaceful area, take a comfortable seat, and concentrate on your breathing or a particular bodily experience.

3. Progressive Muscle Relaxation: A technique called progressive muscle relaxation entails tensing and relaxing various bodily muscle groups. Start by tensing the muscles in your toes and feet, then gradually work your way up to your calves, thighs, abdomen, chest, arms, and finally your face and neck. Hold each muscle contraction for a few seconds, then release and relax completely.

4. Exercise and Physical Activity: Regular exercise is not only beneficial for blood sugar control but also for stress management. Engaging in physical activity can help reduce stress hormones, improve mood, and increase feelings of well-being. Find activities that you enjoy, whether it's walking, jogging, cycling, yoga, or dancing, and make them a regular part of your routine.

5. Healthy Lifestyle Habits: Adopting healthy lifestyle habits such as getting adequate sleep, maintaining a balanced diet, staying hydrated, and limiting caffeine and alcohol intake can help reduce stress levels and support stable blood sugar control.

Aim for seven to nine hours of quality sleep per night and prioritize nutritious foods that fuel your body and mind.

6. Social Support: Seek support from friends, family, or support groups during times of stress. Talking to someone you trust about your feelings and experiences can provide emotional validation, perspective, and encouragement. Surround yourself with positive influences and lean on your support network when needed.

7. Time Management: Being able to prioritize work, create realistic goals, and schedule downtime for rest and self-care are all ways that effective time management can help you feel less stressed. Break tasks into smaller, manageable steps, delegate when possible, and learn to say no to additional responsibilities when you're feeling overwhelmed.

8. Mindful Eating: Practice mindful eating by paying attention to your hunger and fullness cues, savoring each bite, and choosing nourishing foods that support stable blood sugar levels. Avoid eating in front of the TV or computer, and take time to appreciate the flavors, textures, and aromas of your meals.

Incorporating Stress Management into Your Daily Routine

Integrating stress management techniques into your daily routine can help you build resilience, improve blood sugar control, and enhance overall well-being. Experiment with different techniques to find what works best for you, and make a commitment to prioritize stress management as an essential component of your health regimen. Remember that consistency is key, and small, consistent actions can lead to significant improvements over time.

In conclusion, stress management is crucial for maintaining stable blood sugar levels and overall health. By incorporating stress management techniques into your daily routine, you can reduce the impact of stress on blood sugar, improve insulin sensitivity, and reduce the risk of developing type 2 diabetes. Whether it's deep breathing exercises, mindfulness meditation, progressive muscle relaxation, or regular physical activity, find strategies that resonate with you and make them a regular part of your lifestyle. By taking proactive steps to manage stress, you can empower yourself to take control of your health and well-being, one breath at a time.

Quality Sleep and Its Impact on Blood Sugar Levels

Quality sleep is essential for overall health and well-being, and it plays a significant role in regulating blood sugar levels. In this chapter, we will delve into the importance of quality sleep and its profound impact on blood sugar control, drawing from scientific research and personal experiences to highlight key insights and practical strategies.

Understanding the Link Between Sleep and Blood Sugar

Quality sleep is intricately linked to various physiological processes, including glucose metabolism and insulin sensitivity. During sleep, the body undergoes essential repair and regeneration processes, and disruptions to this natural cycle can have adverse effects on blood sugar regulation. Lack of sleep or poor-quality sleep can lead to insulin resistance, impaired glucose tolerance, and increased risk of type 2 diabetes.

My Personal Experience

Reflecting on my own journey, I've experienced firsthand the effects of sleep deprivation on blood sugar levels. During periods of inadequate sleep, I noticed fluctuations in my glucose readings and struggled to maintain stable levels throughout the day. However, by prioritizing quality sleep and implementing strategies to improve sleep hygiene, I was able to better manage my blood sugar and overall health. These personal experiences have underscored the importance of quality sleep in blood sugar control.

The Importance of Sleep Hygiene

1. Consistent Sleep Schedule: Even on weekends, stick to a regular sleep routine by going to bed and waking up at the same times each day. This encourages improved sleep quality and enables your body's internal clock to be more balanced.

2. Create a Relaxing Bedtime Routine: To tell your body it's time to wind down and get ready for sleep, establish a calming nighttime ritual. This could involve doing things like reading, having a warm bath, meditating, or deep breathing, or just listening to relaxing music

3. Optimize Your Sleep Environment: Establish an atmosphere that encourages relaxation and restful sleep. Keep your bedroom cool, dark, and quiet, and invest in a comfortable mattress and pillows to support proper alignment and comfort.

4. Limit Screen Time Before Bed: Minimize exposure to screens, such as smartphones, tablets, computers, and televisions, in the hour leading up to bedtime. The blue light emitted by electronic devices can interfere with melatonin production and disrupt sleep patterns.

5. Watch Your Caffeine and Alcohol Intake: Limit consumption of caffeine and alcohol, especially in the hours leading up to bedtime. Both substances can disrupt sleep patterns and interfere with the quality of your rest.

6. Manage Stress and Anxiety: Practice stress-reduction techniques such as mindfulness meditation, deep breathing exercises, or progressive muscle relaxation to help alleviate stress and promote relaxation before bedtime.

7. Exercise Regularly: Engage in regular physical activity during the day, as it can help improve sleep quality and duration. On the other hand, stay away from strenuous exercise right before bed as it could keep you from falling asleep.

The Impact of Sleep Disorders on Blood Sugar

1. Insomnia: Insomnia, characterized by difficulty falling asleep or staying asleep, can disrupt normal sleep patterns and lead to inadequate restorative sleep. Chronic insomnia is associated with increased risk of insulin resistance and type 2 diabetes.

2. Sleep Apnea: Sleep apnea is a sleep disorder characterized by pauses in breathing during sleep, often accompanied by loud snoring and daytime fatigue. Untreated sleep apnea can contribute to insulin resistance, glucose intolerance, and elevated blood sugar levels.

In conclusion, quality sleep is essential for regulating blood sugar levels and supporting overall health and well-being. By prioritizing sleep hygiene and adopting healthy sleep habits, you can improve sleep quality and duration, enhance insulin sensitivity, and reduce the risk of developing type 2 diabetes. Whether it's maintaining a consistent sleep schedule, creating a relaxing bedtime routine, optimizing your sleep environment, or seeking treatment for sleep disorders, investing in quality sleep is one of the most valuable investments you can make for your health. By nurturing a healthy sleep environment and prioritizing restorative sleep, you can empower yourself to take control of your blood sugar and live a happier, healthier life.

Strategies for Long-Term Success and Maintenance

Achieving success in managing blood sugar levels is a commendable accomplishment, but maintaining long-term success requires commitment, consistency, and strategic planning. In this chapter, we will explore effective strategies for sustaining your progress and achieving lasting results in blood sugar control, drawing from both scientific research and personal experiences to provide actionable insights and guidance.

Understanding the Importance of Long-Term Success

Long-term success in managing blood sugar levels is essential for preventing complications associated with diabetes and promoting overall health and well-being. While short-term changes may yield immediate benefits, sustained efforts are necessary to maintain optimal blood sugar control and reduce the risk of long-term complications.

My Personal Experience

Reflecting on my own journey, I've encountered various challenges and setbacks in managing blood sugar levels over the long term. However, by adopting specific strategies and making lifestyle modifications, I've been able to sustain my progress and achieve lasting success in blood sugar control. These personal experiences have shaped my understanding of the importance of long-term maintenance and inspired me to share these strategies with others.

Strategies for Long-Term Success

1. Establish Realistic Goals: Set realistic and achievable goals for blood sugar management, taking into account your individual circumstances, preferences, and health goals. Divide more ambitious objectives into more doable steps, and acknowledge each accomplishment as it occurs.

2. Create a Sustainable Plan: Develop a sustainable plan for managing blood sugar levels that includes healthy eating habits, regular physical activity, stress management techniques, and consistent monitoring of blood sugar readings. Focus on creating habits that you can maintain over the long term rather than resorting to quick fixes or fad diets.

3. Monitor Blood Sugar Regularly: Regular monitoring of blood sugar levels is essential for identifying patterns, trends, and fluctuations that may require adjustments to your treatment plan or lifestyle habits. Keep track of your blood sugar

readings using a blood glucose meter or continuous glucose monitoring system, and work closely with your healthcare team to interpret and act on the results.

4. Adopt a Balanced Diet: Focus on adopting a balanced and nutritious diet that includes a variety of fruits, vegetables, whole grains, lean proteins, and healthy fats. Aim to incorporate foods with a low glycemic index to help stabilize blood sugar levels and minimize fluctuations throughout the day. Avoid overly restrictive diets or extreme dietary changes that are difficult to maintain over the long term.

5. Engage in Regular Physical Activity: Incorporate regular physical activity into your routine, aiming for at least 150 minutes of moderate-intensity aerobic exercise per week, along with strength training exercises two or more days per week. Find activities that you enjoy and make them a regular part of your lifestyle to promote long-term adherence.

6. Practice Stress Management: Implement stress management techniques such as deep breathing exercises, mindfulness meditation, progressive muscle relaxation, or yoga to reduce stress levels and promote overall well-being. Make self-care activities that support your relaxation, rejuvenation, and optimistic attitude a priority.

7. Seek Support and Accountability: Surround yourself with a supportive network of friends, family, healthcare professionals, or support groups who can provide encouragement, guidance, and accountability on your journey to long-term blood sugar control. Share your goals, challenges, and successes with others, and lean on them for support when needed.

8. Stay Informed and Educated: Stay informed about the latest developments in diabetes management, blood sugar control, and lifestyle interventions by seeking reliable sources of information, attending educational workshops or seminars, and staying connected with your healthcare team. Empower yourself with knowledge and understanding to make informed decisions about your health.

Achieving long-term success and maintenance in blood sugar control requires dedication, perseverance, and a comprehensive approach to health and wellness. By establishing realistic goals, creating a sustainable plan, monitoring blood sugar regularly, adopting a balanced diet, engaging in regular physical activity, practicing stress management techniques, seeking support and accountability, and staying informed and educated, you can empower yourself to sustain your progress and achieve lasting results in blood sugar control.

Remember that small, consistent actions taken over time can lead to significant improvements in your health and well-being. With determination, resilience, and the right strategies in place, you can thrive in your journey to long-term blood sugar management.

CHAPTER 4:

BLOOD SUGAR DIET SUCCESS STORIES

Real-Life Success Stories and Testimonials on Blood Sugar Diet

Real-life success stories and testimonials serve as powerful inspirations for individuals seeking to manage their blood sugar levels and improve their overall health. In this chapter, we will showcase a collection of real-life success stories and testimonials from individuals who have experienced significant improvements in their blood sugar control through the adoption of a blood sugar diet. These stories offer valuable insights, motivation, and encouragement for readers embarking on their own journey to better health.

My Personal Experience

As I embarked on my journey to manage my blood sugar levels and improve my health, I encountered numerous challenges and setbacks. However, through perseverance, dedication, and the adoption of a blood sugar diet, I was able to achieve significant improvements in my blood sugar control and overall well-being. My personal experience serves as a testament to the effectiveness of lifestyle interventions in managing blood sugar levels and inspires me to share the stories of others who have experienced similar transformations.

Success Story 1: Sarah's Journey to Blood Sugar Control

Sarah, a 45-year-old mother of two, struggled with uncontrolled blood sugar levels for years. Despite taking medication and following dietary recommendations, her blood sugar readings remained consistently high, putting her at risk for diabetes complications. Frustrated and discouraged, Sarah decided to take matters into her own hands and adopted a blood sugar diet focused on whole foods, lean proteins, and low-glycemic carbohydrates. Within weeks, Sarah noticed significant improvements in her blood sugar levels, with readings consistently within the target range. Encouraged by her progress, Sarah continued to prioritize healthy eating habits and regular exercise, leading to sustained improvements in her blood sugar control and overall health.

Success Story 2: John's Transformation Through Lifestyle Changes

John, a 55-year-old office worker, was diagnosed with prediabetes after routine blood tests revealed elevated fasting blood sugar levels. Concerned about his health and determined to avoid progressing to type 2 diabetes, John decided to make significant lifestyle changes. He started by revamping his diet, cutting out sugary drinks, refined carbohydrates, and processed foods, and replacing them with whole grains, vegetables, and lean proteins. John also committed to a regular exercise routine, incorporating brisk walks, strength training, and yoga into his weekly schedule. Over time, John's efforts paid off, and his blood sugar levels gradually returned to normal range. Today, John maintains his healthy lifestyle habits and feels better than ever, with improved energy levels, mood, and overall well-being.

Success Story 3: Maria's Journey to Reversing Type 2 Diabetes

Maria, a 60-year-old retiree, was diagnosed with type 2 diabetes and prescribed multiple medications to manage her blood sugar levels. Dissatisfied with relying on medication to control her condition, Maria sought alternative solutions and discovered the transformative power of a blood sugar diet. With guidance from her healthcare team and support from her family, Maria overhauled her diet, focusing on whole, unprocessed foods and limiting added sugars and refined carbohydrates. She also committed to regular physical activity, incorporating daily walks and strength training sessions into her routine. As a result of her efforts, Maria experienced significant improvements in her blood sugar control, leading to the gradual reduction of her medication doses. Today, Maria proudly shares her journey to reversing type 2 diabetes through lifestyle changes, serving as an inspiration to others facing similar challenges.

Success Story 4: James' Triumph Over Diabetes Complications

James, a 50-year-old father of three, struggled with uncontrolled type 2 diabetes for years, experiencing a myriad of complications, including neuropathy, retinopathy, and cardiovascular issues. Determined to reclaim his health and improve his quality of life, James committed to a comprehensive approach to blood sugar management, incorporating a blood sugar diet, regular exercise, stress management techniques, and medication adherence into his daily routine. Despite facing numerous obstacles along the way, including setbacks and relapses, James persevered, drawing strength from his family and the support of his healthcare team. Over time, James experienced remarkable improvements in his blood sugar control, with reductions in HbA1c levels and a resolution of diabetes-related complications. Today, James lives an active, fulfilling life, empowered by his journey to triumph over diabetes and regain control of his health.

In conclusion, these real-life success stories and testimonials underscore the transformative power of lifestyle interventions in managing blood sugar levels and improving overall health. From Sarah's journey to blood sugar control through dietary changes to John's transformation through lifestyle modifications, and Maria's triumph over type 2 diabetes complications to James' perseverance in overcoming adversity, these stories serve as powerful reminders of the potential for positive change through dedication, commitment, and resilience. By sharing these stories, we aim to inspire and motivate others embarking on their own journey to better blood sugar control and enhanced well-being. Together, we can empower individuals to take charge of their health and achieve lasting success in blood sugar management.

Challenges and Solutions: Overcoming Roadblocks on Blood Sugar Diet

Embarking on a blood sugar diet journey can be empowering and transformative, but it's not without its challenges. In this chapter, we'll explore common roadblocks individuals may encounter while following a blood sugar diet and provide practical solutions to overcome them. Drawing from both scientific research and personal experiences, we'll address key challenges and offer actionable strategies to help readers navigate their journey to better blood sugar control.

My Personal Experience

As I embarked on my own blood sugar diet journey, I encountered various challenges that tested my resolve and commitment. From navigating social situations to overcoming cravings and managing stress, each obstacle presented an opportunity for growth and learning. Through trial and error, I discovered effective strategies to overcome these challenges and stay on track with my blood sugar diet. My personal experiences have shaped my understanding of the common roadblocks individuals may face and inspired me to share practical solutions with others embarking on their own journey to better health.

Challenge 1: Social Situations and Peer Pressure

One of the most significant challenges individuals may face on a blood sugar diet is navigating social situations and peer pressure. Whether it's attending social gatherings, dining out with friends, or family events, the temptation to indulge in high-sugar, high-carb foods can be overwhelming.

Solution: Prepare in advance by communicating your dietary needs and preferences to friends and family members. Offer to bring a healthy dish to social gatherings to ensure there are options available that align with your blood sugar diet. Focus on socializing and enjoying the company of others rather than solely on the food. Practice assertiveness and learn to say no politely when offered foods that don't align with your dietary goals.

Challenge 2: Cravings and Temptations

Cravings for sugary and high-carb foods can pose a significant challenge for individuals following a blood sugar diet. These cravings can be triggered by various factors, including stress, emotional eating, and environmental cues.

Solution: Identify the root cause of your cravings and develop strategies to address them. Practice mindful eating by paying attention to hunger and fullness cues and choosing nourishing foods that satisfy your cravings in a healthier way. Keep healthy snacks on hand to curb cravings and prevent impulsive eating. Engage in stress-reduction techniques such as deep breathing, meditation, or yoga to manage stress and reduce emotional eating.

Challenge 3: Time Constraints and Busy Lifestyles

Many individuals cite time constraints and busy lifestyles as barriers to following a blood sugar diet effectively. Balancing work, family responsibilities, and other commitments can make it challenging to prioritize healthy eating and meal preparation.

Solution: Plan and prep meals in advance to save time and streamline your cooking process. Batch, cook and freeze meals for busy days when you don't have time to cook. Invest in time-saving kitchen gadgets such as a slow cooker or Instant Pot to make meal preparation more efficient. Prioritize self-care and make time for activities that promote relaxation and stress management, such as exercise, meditation, or hobbies.

Challenge 4: Plateauing and Lack of Progress

Plateauing and lack of progress can be discouraging for individuals following a blood sugar diet, especially if they've seen initial improvements in blood sugar control but then hit a plateau.

Solution: Reevaluate your dietary habits and lifestyle choices to identify areas for improvement.

Experiment with different meal combinations, portion sizes, and macronutrient ratios to see what works best for your body. Incorporate variety into your diet to prevent boredom and keep your taste buds stimulated. Stay patient and persistent, and remember that progress may not always be linear.

Challenge 5: Emotional Eating and Stress

Emotional eating and stress can sabotage efforts to follow a blood sugar diet, leading to overeating and poor food choices.

Solution: Develop healthy coping mechanisms for managing stress and emotions, such as journaling, practicing relaxation techniques, or seeking support from friends or a therapist. Find alternative ways to cope with stress and emotional triggers, such as going for a walk, listening to music, or engaging in a hobby. Practice self-compassion and forgiveness, and don't be too hard on yourself if you slip up occasionally.

Challenge 6: Lack of Support and Accountability

Lack of support and accountability can make it challenging to stay motivated and committed to a blood sugar diet, especially if friends or family members aren't on board with your dietary goals.

Solution: Seek support from like-minded individuals who share similar health goals and values. Join online communities, support groups, or forums where you can connect with others following a blood sugar diet. Enlist the support of friends and family members by communicating your goals and asking for their encouragement and assistance. Consider working with a registered dietitian or health coach who can provide guidance, accountability, and personalized support.

In conclusion, overcoming roadblocks on a blood sugar diet requires awareness, perseverance, and a proactive approach. By acknowledging common challenges such as social situations, cravings, time constraints, plateauing, emotional eating, and lack of support, individuals can develop effective strategies to navigate their journey to better blood sugar control successfully. By incorporating practical solutions and staying committed to their dietary goals, individuals can overcome obstacles and achieve lasting success in managing their blood sugar levels and improving their overall health and well-being. Remember that progress may not always be linear, and setbacks are a natural part of the journey. Stay resilient, stay focused, and keep moving forward toward your health goals.

CHAPTER 5:

EXPERT ADVICE AND INSIGHTS ON BLOOD SUGAR DIET SOLUTION

In this chapter, we'll delve into expert advice and insights on the blood sugar diet solution. Drawing from the expertise of healthcare professionals, nutritionists, and personal experiences, we'll explore practical tips and strategies to help you effectively manage your blood sugar levels and improve your overall health.

Expert Tips And Insights: Understanding the Blood Sugar Diet

Before we delve into expert advice, let's ensure we're on the same page regarding the blood sugar diet. This dietary approach focuses on stabilizing blood sugar levels by prioritizing whole, nutrient-dense foods while minimizing the intake of sugars and refined carbohydrates. By adopting this approach, individuals can promote better blood sugar control, enhance insulin sensitivity, and reduce the risk of metabolic disorders such as type 2 diabetes and obesity.

Expert Tip 1: Embrace Whole, Unprocessed Foods

One of the fundamental principles of the blood sugar diet is to prioritize whole, unprocessed foods. Fruits, vegetables, whole grains, lean meats, and healthy fats are a few of these. By centering your diet around these nutritious options, you provide your body with essential vitamins, minerals, and antioxidants while minimizing the intake of empty calories and harmful additives.

Expert Tip 2: Mind Your Portions

While the quality of your food choices matters, so does the quantity. Paying attention to portion sizes can help prevent overeating and promote better blood sugar control. Aim to fill half your plate with vegetables, one-quarter with lean protein, and one-quarter with whole grains or starchy vegetables. This balanced approach ensures you're getting a variety of nutrients without overloading on carbohydrates.

Expert Tip 3: Choose Low-Glycemic Foods

Selecting carbohydrates with a low glycemic index (GI) can help stabilize blood sugar levels and prevent sharp spikes and crashes. Low-GI foods are digested and absorbed more slowly, resulting in a gradual rise in blood sugar levels. Examples include legumes, whole grains, non-starchy vegetables, and certain fruits like berries. Incorporating these foods into your meals can promote sustained energy levels and reduce the risk of blood sugar fluctuations.

Expert Tip 4: Be Mindful of Added Sugars

Added sugars hide in many processed foods and beverages, contributing to excess calorie intake and adverse effects on blood sugar levels. To minimize your consumption of added sugars, read food labels carefully and opt for products with little to no added sugars. Choose whole, unprocessed foods whenever possible and use natural sweeteners like fruit or small amounts of honey or maple syrup sparingly.

Expert Tip 5: Prioritize Regular Physical Activity

Physical activity plays a crucial role in managing blood sugar levels and promoting overall health. Aim for at least 150 minutes of moderate-intensity aerobic exercise per week, along with strength training exercises two or more days per week. Find activities you enjoy and incorporate them into your daily routine to make exercise a sustainable and enjoyable habit.

Expert Tip 6: Monitor Your Blood Sugar Levels

Regular monitoring of blood sugar levels is essential for understanding how your dietary and lifestyle choices impact your metabolic health. Work with your healthcare provider to establish target blood sugar ranges and develop a monitoring schedule that works for you. Keep a log of your blood sugar readings, along with details about your meals, physical activity, medications, and any other relevant factors.

Expert Tip 7: Seek Support and Accountability

Embarking on a blood sugar diet journey can be challenging, but you don't have to go it alone. Seek support from friends, family members, or healthcare professionals who can offer encouragement, guidance, and accountability. Joining a support group or online community can also provide valuable resources and connections with others who are on a similar journey.

Personal Experience

As I embarked on my journey to better blood sugar control, I encountered various challenges and uncertainties. However, by incorporating expert advice and insights into my daily routine, I was able to make meaningful progress towards my health goals. Embracing whole, unprocessed foods, minding my portions, choosing low-glycemic options, being mindful of added sugars, prioritizing physical activity, monitoring my blood sugar levels, and seeking support and accountability were key factors in my success. In conclusion, expert advice and insights on the blood sugar diet solution provide valuable guidance and support for individuals looking to improve their metabolic health. By incorporating these practical tips and strategies into your daily routine, you can effectively manage your blood sugar levels, enhance insulin sensitivity, and reduce the risk of metabolic disorders. Remember to approach your dietary and lifestyle changes with patience, persistence, and a commitment to your health goals. With dedication and determination, you can achieve lasting improvements in blood sugar control and enjoy a healthier, happier life.

Common Questions about the Blood Sugar Diet

Navigating the complexities of a blood sugar diet can raise numerous questions for individuals seeking to improve their health and manage their blood sugar levels effectively. In this chapter, we will address some of the most common questions about the blood sugar diet, drawing from scientific research and personal experiences to provide clear and informative answers.

My Personal Experience

As I embarked on my journey to better blood sugar control, I encountered various questions and uncertainties about the blood sugar diet. Through research, experimentation, and guidance from healthcare professionals, I gained valuable insights into the principles and practices of the blood sugar diet. My personal experiences have equipped me with the knowledge and understanding to address common questions and provide practical guidance to others on their journey to improved health.

Question 1: What is the Blood Sugar Diet?

The blood sugar diet is a dietary approach designed to regulate blood sugar levels and promote overall health and well-being. It focuses on consuming whole, unprocessed foods that are low in sugar and carbohydrates while emphasizing nutrient-dense options such as vegetables, fruits, lean proteins, and healthy fats. By prioritizing foods that have a minimal impact on blood sugar levels, the diet aims to stabilize glucose levels, improve insulin sensitivity, and reduce the risk of developing type 2 diabetes and other related health conditions.

Question 2: How Does the Blood Sugar Diet Work?

The blood sugar diet works by controlling the intake of carbohydrates, particularly those that are high in sugars and refined grains. By reducing the consumption of these foods, the diet helps prevent rapid spikes and crashes in blood sugar levels, which can lead to insulin resistance and other metabolic disturbances. Additionally, focusing on nutrient-dense, whole foods helps support overall health and provides essential vitamins, minerals, and antioxidants that contribute to optimal blood sugar control and metabolic function.

Question 3: What Foods Should I Eat on the Blood Sugar Diet?

On the blood sugar diet, it's recommended to prioritize whole, unprocessed foods that are low in sugars and carbohydrates. This includes plenty of vegetables, fruits (in moderation), lean proteins such as poultry, fish, eggs, and tofu, and healthy fats like avocados, nuts, seeds, and olive oil. Foods with a low glycemic index, such as legumes, whole grains, and non-starchy vegetables, are also encouraged as they have a minimal impact on blood sugar levels.

Question 4: Are There Foods to Avoid on the Blood Sugar Diet?

While following the blood sugar diet, it's advisable to limit or avoid foods that are high in sugars, refined grains, and processed ingredients. This includes sugary beverages, sweets, pastries, white bread, sugary cereals, and packaged snacks. Additionally, it's important to moderate intake of starchy vegetables, fruits with high sugar content, and carbohydrate-rich foods that can cause rapid spikes in blood sugar levels.

Question 5: Can I Lose Weight on the Blood Sugar Diet?

Many individuals experience weight loss as a secondary benefit of following the blood sugar diet. By focusing on whole, nutrient-dense foods and controlling carbohydrate intake, the diet can help regulate appetite, promote satiety, and support sustainable weight loss. Additionally, stabilizing blood sugar levels can reduce cravings for sugary and high-calorie foods, making it easier to adhere to a healthy eating plan and achieve long-term weight management goals.

Question 6: Is the Blood Sugar Diet Safe for Everyone?

The blood sugar diet is generally considered safe for most individuals, but it's important to consult with a healthcare professional before making any significant dietary changes, especially if you have pre-existing health conditions or are taking medications. People with diabetes, in particular, should work closely with their healthcare team to ensure that the diet is appropriate for their individual needs and medical history.

Question 7: How Can I Get Started on the Blood Sugar Diet?

Getting started on the blood sugar diet is relatively straightforward. Begin by familiarizing yourself with the principles of the diet and gradually make small changes to your eating habits. Start by incorporating more whole, nutrient-dense foods into your meals and reducing your intake of sugary and processed foods. Experiment with new recipes, meal ideas, and food combinations to keep your meals interesting and satisfying. Consider seeking support from a registered dietitian or health coach who can provide personalized guidance and support as you embark on your journey to better blood sugar control.

The blood sugar diet offers a practical and effective approach to managing blood sugar levels and improving overall health. By prioritizing whole, nutrient-dense foods and controlling carbohydrate intake, individuals can stabilize blood sugar levels, reduce the risk of metabolic disturbances, and achieve long-term health and wellness. By addressing common questions and providing clear, informative answers, we hope to empower readers with the knowledge and understanding they need to embark on their own journey to better blood sugar control and improved quality of life. Remember to consult with a healthcare professional before making any significant dietary changes, and approach your journey with patience, persistence, and a commitment to your health goals.

CONCLUSION

Embracing the Journey to Better Health

As we come to the end of our exploration into the blood sugar diet solution, I find myself reflecting on the transformative journey we've embarked upon together. Throughout this book, we've delved deep into the intricacies of blood sugar regulation, dietary choices, lifestyle habits, and the profound impact they have on our health and well-being. We've uncovered insights, strategies, and practical tips to empower us on our path to better health. And as we bid farewell to these pages, I am filled with a sense of fulfillment and motivation, knowing that our journey has only just begun.

At the heart of our exploration lies a central message: the power to transform our health resides within each of us. It's about recognizing that every choice we make – from the foods we eat to the activities we engage in – has the potential to shape our health outcomes. It's about embracing a holistic approach to health that nurtures not just our bodies, but also our minds and spirits. And it's about understanding that true wellness is a journey, not a destination – a journey that requires dedication, perseverance, and a commitment to lifelong learning and growth.

Throughout this book, we've touched upon key principles and practices that form the foundation of the blood sugar diet solution. We've learned to prioritize whole, nutrient-dense foods, mind our portions, and choose low-glycemic options to stabilize blood sugar levels. We've embraced the importance of regular physical activity, stress management, quality sleep, and maintaining a supportive environment for optimal health. And perhaps most importantly, we've recognized the power of self-awareness, self-care, and self-compassion in nurturing our health and well-being.

But knowledge alone is not enough. It is only through action – through applying the knowledge gained – that we can truly transform our health and our lives. So, as we bid adieu to these pages, I urge you to take the insights, strategies, and practical tips you've acquired and put them into practice in your daily life. Whether it's making small changes to your diet, incorporating more movement into your day, or prioritizing self-care and stress management, every step you take towards better health matters.

And remember, you are not alone on this journey. Seek support from friends, family members, healthcare professionals, or online communities who can offer guidance, encouragement, and accountability along the way. Share your successes and challenges, celebrate your progress, and never hesitate to ask for help when you need it. Together, we can inspire and support each other on our paths to vibrant health and well-being.

As we close this chapter and look towards the future, let us do so with optimism, determination, and a sense of purpose. Let us embrace the journey ahead with open hearts and open minds, knowing that the power to transform our health and our lives lies within us. And let us take action today – right now – to create the vibrant, fulfilling, and healthy life we deserve.

So, dear reader, I invite you to step boldly into the future, armed with the knowledge, insights, and inspiration you've gained from these pages. Embrace the journey, trust in your ability to create positive change, and never forget that the greatest adventure of all is the one that leads us back to ourselves – to our truest, healthiest, and most vibrant selves.

Thank you for joining me on this journey. May your path be filled with joy, vitality, and abundant well-being.

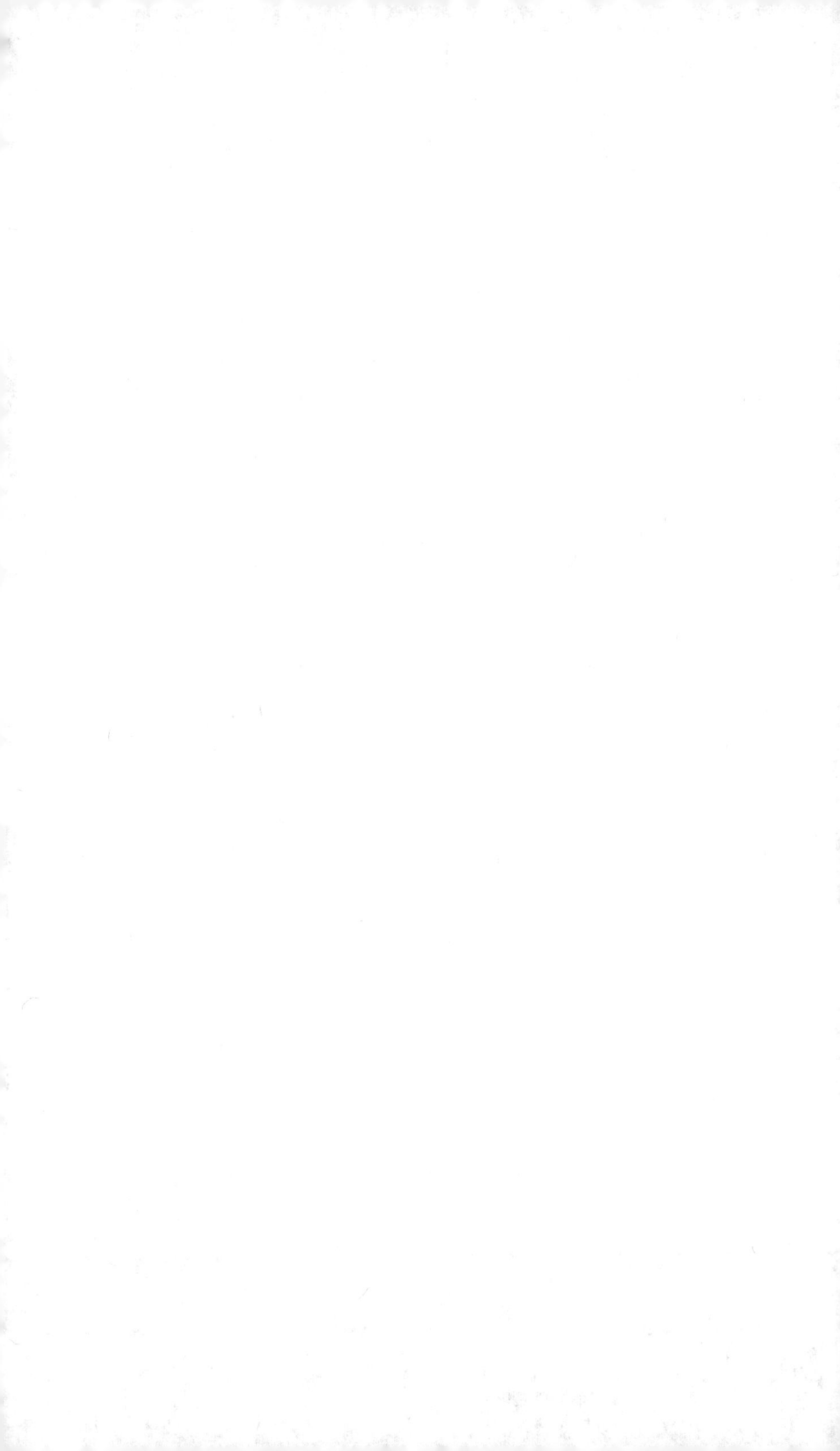

www.ingramcontent.com/pod-product-compliance
Lightning Source LLC
Chambersburg PA
CBHW051833250726
48659CB00005B/1817